YOUR 90-DAY WELLNESS GUIDED
MEDICAL JOURNAL

Jill Johnson

BALANCE LIFE

PHARMACIST BOOK PUBLISHING
Royal Oak, MICHIGAN

YOUR 90-DAY WELLNESS GUIDED
MEDICAL JOURNAL
Published by
BALANCE LIFE PHARMACIST BOOK PUBLISHING
Royal Oak, Michigan
Admin@balanceliferx.com

Jill Johnson, Publisher
Yvonne Rose/Quality Press, Book Packager

ISBN #: 979-8-3495-3712-7

I DEDICATE THIS JOURNAL TO
MONA CHADWICK

THIS JOURNAL BELONGS TO:

____

Table of Contents

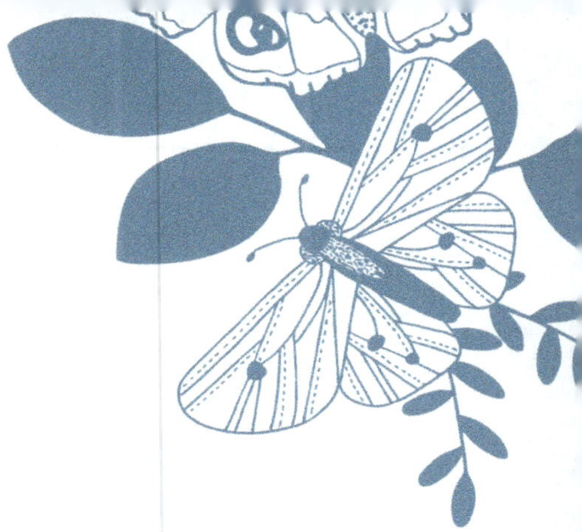

WELCOME TO YOUR HEALTH JOURNAL

"We recognizes that patients have a unique understanding of their own health, symptoms, and how they feel."

This journal is here to support you. Whether you're tracking symptoms, preparing for appointments, or reflecting on your wellness goals, this is your safe space to stay organized and be heard.

Here, we believe your story, your intuition, and your experience matter. You're not alone on this journey —and this journal is your companion to help you advocate for the care you deserve.

"

This Journal Is Yours!!

**Be consistent when possible.
You don't need to fill every box.
This is your place to improve your outcomes and be seen and heard as you move through your healthcare journey.
Allow this journal be that for you.**

"

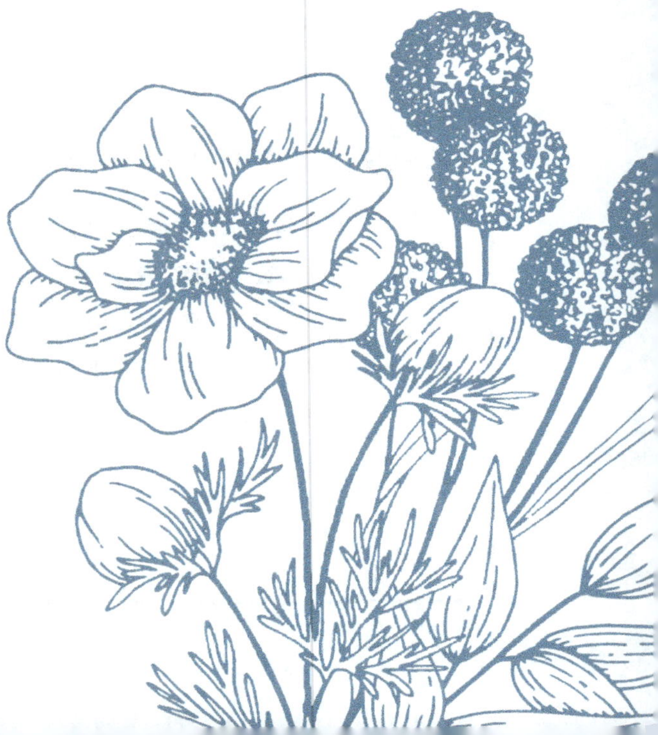

How to

USE THIS JOURNAL

A practical tool for staying organized, knowledgeable and confident in your healthcare journey.

1 Document What You Experience

Use this journal to jot down what you're noticing in your body—symptoms, mood changes, energy shifts, or anything that feels off. You don't have to figure it out on your own, but writing it down as it happens gives you a clearer picture over time and ensures nothing important gets forgotten when it's time to talk with your provider.

2 Track Appointments, Labs & Treatments

Healthcare can be hard to manage when you're juggling multiple appointments, test results, and treatment plans. This journal helps you keep everything in one place—record dates, results, provider notes, and follow-ups so you have an accurate and accessible record of your care history.

3 Prepare Questions Ahead of Time

It's easy to get overwhelmed or forget what you meant to ask once you're in the exam room. Use this journal to write out your questions in advance so you feel confident and prepared. Whether it's about symptoms, medication side effects, or treatment options, bringing clear questions into the room helps you get the answers you need.

...CONTINUED: HOW TO USE THIS JOURNAL

4 Reflect on Your Healing Process

Healing is more than managing symptoms—it's about recognizing your progress and reconnecting with your goals. This journal invites you to reflect on how you're feeling overall, what's improved, what's challenging, and what you hope to shift moving forward, so you stay connected to your whole self—not just your diagnosis.

5 What to Bring With You to Appointments

This journal can be your voice when you're tired, overwhelmed, or unsure what to say. Bring it with you to appointments so you can reference your notes, stay focused during conversations, and even share your entries directly with your provider if needed. You don't have to remember everything—just bring your journal.

> "Good health and good sense are two of life's greatest blessings."
> – Publilius Syrus

Why Doctor-Patient

RELATIONSHIPS MATTER

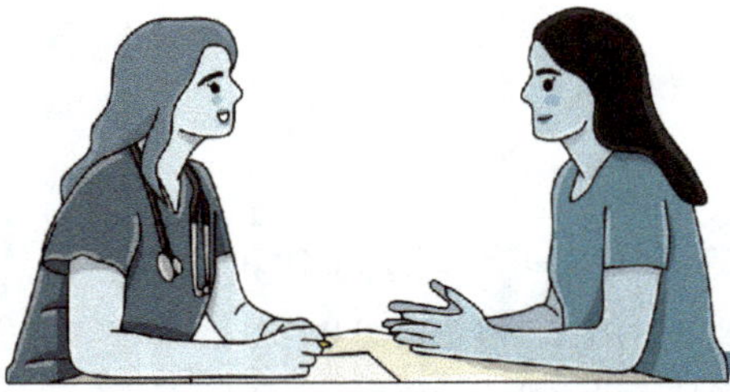

Your care is a partnership—not a one-way street.

A strong relationship with your doctor is one of the most powerful tools in your healing. When a provider truly listens, respects your experience, and includes you in decisions, care becomes collaborative—not just clinical.

You know your body best. That insight matters. This journal helps you come to appointments prepared—with your symptoms, your questions, and your goals—so you can communicate clearly and confidently.

Even in rushed or complex healthcare systems, your preparation helps shift the dynamic. It reminds everyone in the room that your voice belongs in your care.

> **"The best medicine starts with listening."**

Let this journal support you in speaking up, staying organized, and getting the care you deserve.

Before
YOUR APPOINTMENT

Taking just a few minutes to prepare can make your visit smoother, more productive, and less stressful.

☐ **Write down 2–3 main concerns**

Think about the biggest things you want to bring up. Keeping it focused helps your provider understand your priorities.

☐ **List any new symptoms and when they started**

Include how long you've had the symptom, how often it happens, and anything that makes it better or worse.

☐ **Bring a list of medications and supplements**

Include the name, dosage, and how often you take them—even vitamins and herbal remedies. This prevents interactions and keeps your care safe.

☐ **Don't forget to ask your questions**

Jot down your questions in advance. Keep the journal open during your appointment so you don't forget anything important.

☐ **Take notes or bring a support person**

Ask a friend or loved one to come if you feel overwhelmed. If you're solo, use this journal to take notes—it helps you remember instructions and follow-up steps later.

Getting

STARTED

WHY I"M USING THIS JOURNAL?

Take a moment to reflect on what brought you here—what you're seeking and what you're ready to explore.

MY WELLNESS GOALS THIS YEAR

These can be big or small—emotional, physical, spiritual, or lifestyle-related. Your goals are yours alone.

"Progress, not perfection. You're already doing the work."

IN CASE OF EMERGENCY TAKE YOUR HEALTH JOURNAL

Your Essential Guide for Navigating Emergencies

Your health journal isn't just for daily notes—it's your essential guide to staying prepared in emergencies.
Life is unpredictable, and when crises strike, having the right information at your fingertips can help you act with clarity and confidence. This journal is designed to equip you with critical details that matter most when time is short. Whether you're facing a natural disaster, medical emergency, or other unexpected situations, this resource helps ensure that you and your loved ones are ready to respond quickly and effectively.

Let this journal be your trusted companion in times of need.

Inside, you'll find essential sections including:

- **Medical Emergencies:** Step-by-step responses to urgent situations.
- **Symptoms to Watch For**: Know the signs that require immediate action.
- **Emergency Contacts:** A dedicated space for doctors, caregivers, and loved ones.
- **Unexpected Situations:** Real-life scenarios with preparedness tips for your family.
- **Resources:** Tools and references to support your emergency plan.

Legal & Medical Documents Checklist:

- Name and contact of your attorney
- Location of key documents (include copies)
- Birth certificate
- Blood type
- Advance medical directive: A legal document stating what treatments you do or don't want if you become incapacitated, and who is authorized to make decisions on your behalf.

> **"Stay prepared, stay safe, and know that this guide is here to support you through any emergency."**

EMERGENCY CONTACTS

List the people to be contacted in case of an emergency. Include someone close to you and your primary care provider.

Name	Relationship	Phone Number	Alternate Number	Notes (e.g. allergies, preferred hospital)

You can ask your doctor to copy these pages and add them to your record. Tip!

ADVANCE DIRECTIVE

Write down your care wishes now, so your loved ones don't have to guess later.

I______________________ appoint this person to make decisions about my medical care if there ever comes a time when I cannot make those decisions myself. I want the person I have appointed, my doctors, my family and others to be guided by the decisions I have made in the parts of the form that follow.
Name:____
Home telephone: ________________________ Work telephone: ______________________
Address:____

If the person above cannot or will not make decisions for me, I appoint this person:
Name:____
Home telephone: _________________________ Work telephone: ______________________
Address:____

I________________________ have not appointed anyone to make health care decisions for me in this or any other document.

PART 2. MY LIVING WILL

These are my wishes for my future medical care if there ever comes a time when I can't make these decisions for myself.

A. These are my wishes if I have a terminal condition

Life-sustaining treatments:
I________________________ do not want life-sustaining treatment (including CPR) started. If life-sustaining treatments are started, I want them stopped.
I_____ ___________________want the life-sustaining treatments that my doctors think are best for me.

Other wishes
____
____

Note: Please consult a legal advisor or local authority to understand the specific laws and requirements for making an advance directive valid in your state, county, or country.

Tip: Have medical staff make a copy to be placed in your medical records. If you find another form feel free to use that or change the one that I provided.

...CONTINUED: ADVANCE DIRECTIVE

Artificial nutrition and hydration:

I__________________________ do not want artificial nutrition and hydration started if they would be the main treatments keeping me alive. If artificial nutrition and hydration are started, I want them stopped.

I___________________________ want artificial nutrition and hydration even if they are the main treatments keeping me alive.

Other wishes

____

____

Comfort care:

I___________________________ want to be kept as comfortable and free of pain as possible, even if such care prolongs my dying or shortens my life.

Other wishes

____

____

B. These are my wishes if I am ever in a persistent vegetative state

Life-sustaining treatments:

I___________________________ do not want life-sustaining treatments (including CPR) started. If life-sustaining treatments are started, I want them stopped.

I__________________________ I want the life-sustaining treatments that my doctors think are best for me.

Other wishes

____

Artificial nutrition and hydration:

I___________________________ do not want artificial nutrition and hydration started if they would be the main treatments keeping me alive. If artificial nutrition and hydration are started, I want them stopped.

I__________________________want artificial nutrition and hydration even if they are the main treatments keeping me alive.

Other wishes

____

____

Note: Please consult a legal advisor or local authority to understand the specific laws and requirements for making an advance directive valid in your state, county, or country.

Tip: Have medical staff make a copy to be placed in your medical records. If you find another form feel free to use that or change the one that I provided.

...CONTINUED: ADVANCE DIRECTIVE

Comfort care:

I__________________________ want to be kept as comfortable and free of pain as possible, even if such care prolongs my dying or shortens my life.

Other wishes

____

____

C. Other directions

You have the right to be involved in all decisions about your medical care, even those not dealing with terminal conditions or persistent vegetative states. If you have wishes not covered in other parts of this document, please indicate them below.

____

____

____

____

____

____

____

____

____

PART 3. OTHER WISHES

A. Organ donation:

I_______________________ do not wish to donate any of my organs or tissues.

I_______________________ I want to donate all of my organs and tissues.

I_______________________ I only want to donate these organs and tissues:

____

Other wishes

____

____

Note: Please consult a legal advisor or local authority to understand the specific laws and requirements for making an advance directive valid in your state, county, or country.

Tip: Have medical staff make a copy to be placed in your medical records. If you find another form feel free to use that or change the one that I provided.

...CONTINUED: ADVANCE DIRECTIVE

Autopsy:

I__________________________ do not want an autopsy.

I__________________________ I agree to an autopsy if my doctors wish it.

Other wishes

____

____

B. Your witnesses' signatures

I believe the person who has signed this advance directive to be of sound mind, that he/she signed or acknowledged this advance directive in my presence and that he/she appears not to be acting under pressure, duress, fraud or undue influence. I am not a family members, health care team members or beneficiaries of your estate.

Witness #1

Signature ____ Date ____________________

Address____

Witness #2

Signature ____ Date ____________________

Address____

Note: Please consult a legal advisor or local authority to understand the specific laws and requirements for making an advance directive valid in your state, county, or country.

Tip: Have medical staff make a copy to be placed in your medical records. If you find another form feel free to use that or change the one that I provided.

DEFINITIONS TO KNOW

Simple explanations to help you feel more confident and informed as you fill out your advance directive.

- **Advance directive:** a legal form that outlines what kind of care you want —or don't want—if you ever can't make those decisions yourself;
- **Artificial nutrition and hydration:** food and fluids given through a tube when you can't eat or drink by mouth;
- **Autopsy**: a medical exam after death to find out what caused it;
- Comfort care: treatments that ease pain and keep you comfortable, even if they don't cure you;
- **CPR (cardiopulmonary resuscitation)**: an emergency treatment to try to restart your heart or breathing;
- **Durable power of attorney for health care**: a document that names someone to speak for you if you can't make medical decisions yourself;
- **Life-sustaining treatment:** any medical care used to keep you alive, like breathing machines, CPR, or feeding tubes;
- **Living will:** a document that explains what medical care you want if you're unable to speak for yourself;
- **Organ and tissue donation:** allowing your organs or tissues to be used after your death for transplant or medical research;
- **Persistent vegetative state:** a condition where a person is unconscious with no awareness or chance of recovery, even if the body seems awake;
- **Terminal condition:** an illness or injury that can't be cured and is expected to lead to death, even with medical care.

UNEXPECTED SITUATIONS

Emergencies don't wait—but with a little planning, you won't have to panic

Life is full of surprises—some beautiful, some challenging. Whether it's a weather emergency, a sudden evacuation, or an unexpected hospital trip, being prepared helps protect your peace of mind. This page is here to help you think ahead so your family can act with confidence, not chaos.

Real-Life Scenarios + Tips:

🌪 EMERGENCY WEATHER (E.G., HURRICANES, FLOODS, BLIZZARDS)

Prep Tip: Keep your journal in a waterproof pouch along with IDs, prescriptions, and a basic go-bag. Include a small flashlight and contact list.

⚡ POWER OUTAGE / BLACKOUT

Prep Tip: Know where your meds and journal are stored. Keep a charged backup power bank for your phone and write down essential health information in case your devices go down.

🚨 EVACUATION (E.G., WILDFIRE, GAS LEAK)

Prep Tip: Have a checklist ready by the door: medications, medical journal, water, and any urgent care items. Keep copies of advance directives and emergency contacts in your bag.

🚑 SUDDEN HOSPITAL VISIT

Prep Tip: Keep a "grab and go" envelope with your journal, insurance info, ID, current medications, and care team list. Store it in a clearly labeled drawer or bag.

"In the chaos of crisis, calm lives in preparation."

LEGAL & MEDICAL DOCUMENTS CHECKLIST

Keep your most important information and documents in one easy-to-locate place—so you're ready when it matters most.

☑	Document	Notes / Location
☐	Full legal name, address, and contact info	
☐	Emergency contacts list	
☐	Blood type	
☐	Health insurance card / info	
☐	Advance medical directive / living will	
☐	Name and contact of your attorney	
☐	Copy of birth certificate	
☐	Social security card or number	
☐	Copy of ID (driver's license or national ID)	
☐	Health Journal	
☐	Insurance policy numbers and contact info	
☐	Location of key documents	

"You are doing sooo good...you got this!!"

MY MEDICAL SNAPSHOT

"All your important health details, all in one place."

This section is your personal health cheat sheet. Whether you're heading to a new doctor, filling out forms, or just want to keep track of your wellness journey, having your information organized and up to date can make a huge difference.

Think of it as your medical snapshot—clear, current, and always ready when you need it.

> **"Your body holds wisdom, and every detail you track is an act of care. By gathering your story here, you're honoring your journey, advocating for your needs, and reminding yourself that healing starts with being seen and understood. You deserve excellence"**

MY HEALTH OVERVIEW

HOSPITALIZATIONS, CONDITIONS, SURGERIES, ALLERGIES

Condition / Surgery / Allergy	Date/ Diagnosed / Performed	Notes / Severity / Treatment

Use this space to keep track of your medical history. This includes current or past diagnoses, surgeries you've had, and any allergies to medications, foods, or environmental triggers. This information can help doctors make better, safer decisions—especially in emergencies.

You can ask your doctor to copy these pages and add them to your record. Tip!

MEDICATION TRACKER

List all your medications—daily, occasional, OTC, or prescribed.
Keeping this updated helps your care team make safer choices.

Medication:

Frequency:

I use this to treat my

Date	Time	Taken

Medication:

Frequency:

I use this to treat my

Date	Time	Taken

Medication:

Frequency:

I use this to treat my

Date	Time	Taken

"Clarity in your care starts with knowing what you take."

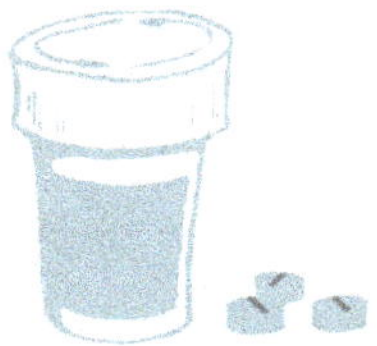

SUPPLEMENT TRACKER

Include vitamins, herbs, or other supplements—even if they're natural, they can interact with medications.

Supplement	Dosage	Frequency	Start Date	End Date	Notes

"Clarity in your care starts with knowing what you take."

Keep track of the professionals supporting your care.

MY CARE TEAM LIST

PROVIDER NAME:

Specialty:

Phone/Email:

Location:

Staff name, RN:

PHARMACY NAME:

ADDRESS:

Phone/Email

INSURANCE ID # **BIN #**

GROUP #

PROVIDER NAME: REMEMBER YOUR DENTIST

Dentist:

Phone/Email:

Location:

"Healing is a team effort—choose people who listen, support, and care."

Keep track of the professionals supporting your care.

MY CARE TEAM LIST

PROVIDER NAME:

Specialty:

Phone/Email

Location:

PROVIDER NAME:

Specialty:

Phone/Email

Location:

PROVIDER NAME:

Specialty:

Phone/Email

Location:

"Healing is a team effort—choose people who listen, support, and care."

Keep track of the professionals supporting your care.

MY CARE TEAM LIST

PROVIDER NAME:

Specialty:

Phone/Email

Location:

PROVIDER NAME:

Specialty:

Phone/Email

Location:

PROVIDER NAME:

Specialty:

Phone/Email

Location:

"Healing is a team effort—choose people who listen, support, and care."

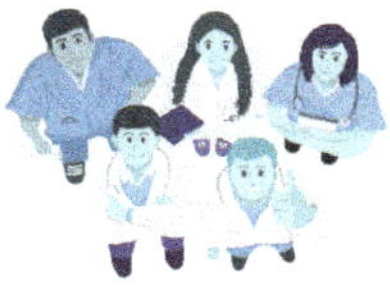

MY GROUPED CARE TEAM CHART

Organize your care team by category

Primary Care Provider(s)

Name	Phone/Email	Location	Notes

Specialists

Name	Phone/Email	Location	Notes

"Healing is a team effort—choose people who listen, support, and care."

...CONTINUED: MY GROUP CARE TEAM CHART

Holistic / Alternative Practitioners

Name	Phone/Email	Location	Notes

Therapists

Name	Phone/Email	Location	Notes

APPOINTMENT PREP

Walk in prepared, walk out empowered.

Appointments can be overwhelming—especially when you're juggling symptoms, questions, and emotions. But being prepared gives you power. It allows you to enter the room with clarity and confidence, knowing you've already thought about what matters most.

This section is your space to plan ahead, voice your concerns, and stay grounded. Whether you're seeing a new provider or following up on care, you deserve to feel heard. Let this page be your anchor.

> **"Advocating for your health starts with knowing what matters to you. When you take a few moments to prepare—gather your thoughts, write down your questions, and name your needs—you give yourself the power to be seen, heard, and cared for with intention."**

APPOINTMENT PLANNER PAGE

Fill this out before each visit to stay focused and ready to speak up.

Date ______________________________

Doctor's Name ______________________________

Clinic ______________________________

Reason for Visit ______________________________

What I Want to Talk About

____

____

____

____

____

Questions I Want to Ask

____

____

____

____

____

What I Want from this Visit

____

____

____

____

____

"When you're prepared, you're powerful."

REMINDER CHECKLIST

Use this list to make sure you have everything you need before you go.

☑

- ☐ Bring this journal
- ☐ Medication & supplement list
- ☐ Lab results or imaging reports (if applicable)
- ☐ Insurance card & ID
- ☐ Referral paperwork (if required)
- ☐ List of allergies
- ☐ Top 3 concerns or symptoms
- ☐ Questions you want to ask
- ☐ A support person (if needed)
- ☐ Something to take notes with pen
- ☐ Hydrate prior to appt. to make labs draws easier
- ☐ Glasses or Hearing Aids

"When you're prepared, you're powerful."

REMINDER TALKING POINTS

Use this list to make sure you cover your talking poinnts

- [x]
- [ ] APPETITE DECREASING
- [ ] SLEEP PATTERN CHANGES
- [ ] DIET CHANGES, DIET MEDICATIONS OR SUPPLEMENTS
- [ ] ILLEGAL DRUGS USED
- [ ] STRESS LEVEL
- [ ] ALCOHOL USE
- [ ] SEXUAL ACTIVITY/PARTNERS
- [ ] FAMILY HISTORY
- [ ] WATER INTAKE DAILY
- [ ] DEPRESSION
- [ ] ______________

"When you're prepared, you're powerful."

APPOINTMENT PLANNER PAGE

Fill this out before each visit to stay focused and ready to speak up.

Date ______________________________

Doctor's Name ______________________________

Clinic ______________________________

Reason for Visit ______________________________

What I Want to Talk About

____

____

____

____

____

Questions I Want to Ask

____

____

____

____

____

What I Want from this Visit

____

____

____

____

____

"When you're prepared, you're powerful."

REMINDER CHECKLIST

Use this list to make sure you have everything you need before you go.

☑

- ☐ Bring this journal
- ☐ Medication & supplement list
- ☐ Lab results or imaging reports (if applicable)
- ☐ Insurance card & ID
- ☐ Referral paperwork (if required)
- ☐ List of allergies
- ☐ Top 3 concerns or symptoms
- ☐ Questions you want to ask
- ☐ A support person (if needed)
- ☐ Something to take notes with pen
- ☐ Hydrate prior to appt. to make labs draws easier
- ☐ Glasses or Hearing Aids

"When you're prepared, you're powerful."

REMINDER TALKING POINTS

Use this list to make sure you cover your talking poinnts

☑

☐ APPETITE DECREASING

☐ SLEEP PATTERN CHANGES

☐ DIET CHANGES, DIET MEDICATION OR SUPPLEMENTS

☐ ILLEGAL DRUGS USE

☐ STRESS LEVEL

☐ ALCOHOL USE

☐ SEXUAL ACTIVITY/PARTNERS

☐ FAMILY HISTORY

☐ WATER INTAKE DAILY

☐ DEPRESSION

☐ ---------------

"When you're prepared, you're powerful."

APPOINTMENT PLANNER PAGE

Fill this out before each visit to stay focused and ready to speak up.

Date ______________________

Doctor's Name ______________________

Clinic ______________________

Reason for Visit ______________________

What I Want to Talk About

____

____

____

____

____

Questions I Want to Ask

____

____

____

____

____

What I Want from this Visit

____

____

____

____

____

"When you're prepared, you're powerful."

REMINDER CHECKLIST

Use this list to make sure you have everything you need before you go.

☑

- ☐ Bring this journal
- ☐ Medication & supplement list
- ☐ Lab results or imaging reports (if applicable)
- ☐ Insurance card & ID
- ☐ Referral paperwork (if required)
- ☐ List of allergies
- ☐ Top 3 concerns or symptoms
- ☐ Questions you want to ask
- ☐ A support person (if needed)
- ☐ Something to take notes with pen
- ☐ Hydrate prior to appt. to make labs draws easier
- ☐ Glasses or Hearing Aids

"When you're prepared, you're powerful."

REMINDER TALKING POINTS

Use this list to make sure you cover your talking poinnts

☑

- ☐ APPETITE DECREASING
- ☐ SLEEP PATTERN CHANGES
- ☐ DIET CHANGES, DIET MEDICATIONS OR SUPPLEMENTS
- ☐ ILLEGAL DRUGS USED
- ☐ STRESS LEVEL
- ☐ ALCOHOL USE
- ☐ SEXUAL ACTIVITY/PARTNERS
- ☐ FAMILY HISTORY
- ☐ WATER INTAKE DAILY
- ☐ DEPRESSION
- ☐ ---------------

"When you're prepared, you're powerful."

Notes

Notes

Notes

AFTER-VISIT NOTES

Keep track of what happened—so you don't have to rely on memory alone.

Sometimes a visit moves fast, or we're handed a lot of information all at once. This page helps you slow it down. Use it to jot down what your provider said, how you felt, and what to follow up on.

Having everything in one place means less stress later—and more confidence moving forward.

> **"Healing doesn't happen all at once—it unfolds in conversations, check-ins, and quiet moments when we give ourselves time to reflect. Every visit is a piece of the puzzle, and writing it down is how we begin to truly see the picture."**

Diagnosis or Outcome

WHAT THE DOCTOR SAID IT WAS

Write down the condition name, diagnosis, or what the provider concluded.

2 Prescriptions or Treatment Plan

WHAT I'M SUPPOSED TO DO NEXT

Medications, lifestyle changes, therapies, etc.

Medication/Treatment	Instructions	Start Date	Notes

3 Follow-Up Steps

NEXT THINGS I NEED TO DO

e.g., schedule a lab, book a follow-up, change routines.

- [ ] ______________________________
- [ ] ______________________________
- [ ] ______________________________
- [ ] ______________________________
- [ ] ______________________________
- [ ] ______________________________
- [ ] ______________________________

"Clarity today makes healing easier tomorrow."

4 Referrals or Tests Ordered

SPECIALISTS, LABS, OR DIAGNOSTICS I WAS REFERRED TO

Include test names, doctor names, and appointment dates if given.

Provider / Test	Reason	Location / Contact	Date / Notes

5 How I Felt After the Visit

EMOTIONAL OR PHYSICAL CHECK-IN

What's Your Mood?

Did you feel heard? Rushed? Relieved? Confused? Tired?

"Clarity today makes healing easier tomorrow."

Reflections

ANYTHING I WANT TO REMEMBER OR BRING UP NEXT TIME

1 Diagnosis or Outcome

WHAT THE DOCTOR SAID IT WAS

Write down the condition name, diagnosis, or what the provider concluded.

"Clarity today makes healing easier tomorrow."

2 Prescriptions or Treatment Plan

WHAT I'M SUPPOSED TO DO NEXT

Medications, lifestyle changes, therapies, etc.

Medication/Treatment	Instructions	Start Date	Notes

3 Follow-Up Steps

NEXT THINGS I NEED TO DO

e.g., schedule a lab, book a follow-up, change routines.

- [ ] ______________________________
- [ ] ______________________________
- [ ] ______________________________
- [ ] ______________________________
- [ ] ______________________________
- [ ] ______________________________
- [ ] ______________________________

"Clarity today makes healing easier tomorrow."

4 Referrals or Tests Ordered

SPECIALISTS, LABS, OR DIAGNOSTICS I WAS REFERRED TO

Include test names, doctor names, and appointment dates if given.

Provider / Test	Reason	Location / Contact	Date / Notes

5 How I Felt After the Visit

EMOTIONAL OR PHYSICAL CHECK-IN

What's Your Mood?

Did you feel heard? Rushed? Relieved? Confused? Tired?

"Clarity today makes healing easier tomorrow."

Reflections

ANYTHING I WANT TO REMEMBER OR BRING UP NEXT TIME

Diagnosis or Outcome

WHAT THE DOCTOR SAID IT WAS

Write down the condition name, diagnosis, or what the provider concluded.

2 Prescriptions or Treatment Plan

WHAT I'M SUPPOSED TO DO NEXT

Medications, lifestyle changes, therapies, etc.

Medication/Treatment	Instructions	Start Date	Notes

3 Follow-Up Steps

NEXT THINGS I NEED TO DO

e.g., schedule a lab, book a follow-up, change routines.

- [ ] ______________________
- [ ] ______________________
- [ ] ______________________
- [ ] ______________________
- [ ] ______________________
- [ ] ______________________
- [ ] ______________________

"Clarity today makes healing easier tomorrow."

4 Referrals or Tests Ordered

SPECIALISTS, LABS, OR DIAGNOSTICS I WAS REFERRED TO

Include test names, doctor names, and appointment dates if given.

Provider / Test	Reason	Location / Contact	Date / Notes

5 How I Felt After the Visit

EMOTIONAL OR PHYSICAL CHECK-IN

Did you feel heard? Rushed? Relieved? Confused? Tired?

What's Your Mood?

"Clarity today makes healing easier tomorrow."

Reflections

ANYTHING I WANT TO REMEMBER OR BRING UP NEXT TIME

LAB RESULTS TRACKER

Track your numbers, notice patterns, and stay informed.

Lab results can feel overwhelming—but they're also powerful clues about your body's inner landscape. This section is designed to help you understand and track your results over time, so you can see the big picture and spot meaningful trends. Whether you're monitoring chronic conditions, healing from illness, or just staying proactive, these pages give you space to stay organized and engaged in your own care.

By recording your labs here, you'll be able to bring clearer questions to your appointments and notice when something shifts. And that kind of awareness? It's a form of advocacy.

> **"Your lab results don't define you—but they do tell a story. When you listen closely, you begin to understand not just what needs healing, but how far you've already come."**

COMMON LAB VALUES (U.S. UNITS)

To offer quick reference ranges for common labs, so the user can compare safely and accurately.

Test	Normal Range	High May Indicate	Low May Indicate
WBC	4.5–11 x10^3/µL	Infection, inflammation	Immune suppression
RBC	4.7–6.1 M/µL (men)	Dehydration, polycythemia	Anemia, blood loss
Hemoglobin	13.8–17.2 g/dL (men)	Lung disease	Anemia
Hematocrit	40.7–50.3% (men)	Dehydration	Blood loss
Platelets	150–450 x10^3/µL	Clotting risk	Bleeding risk
Glucose (fasting)	70–99 mg/dL	Diabetes	Hypoglycemia
A1C	Below 5.7%	Diabetes	Hyperthyroidism
TSH	0.4–4.0 mIU/L	Hypothyroidism	Low blood sugar episodes
Vitamin D	30–50 ng/mL	Toxicity	Deficiency
B12	200–900 pg/mL	Supplement overdose	Fatigue, nerve issues

"When you know your numbers, you know your body."

MY PERSONAL LAB RESULTS TRACKER

Include vitamins, herbs, or other supplements—even if they're natural,
They can interact with medications.

Date	labs	Result	Normal Range	Notes

"When you know your numbers, you know your body."

MY PERSONAL LAB RESULTS TRACKER

Include vitamins, herbs, or other supplements—even if they're natural,
They can interact with medications.

Date	labs	Result	Normal Range	Notes

"When you know your numbers, you know your body."

Your Journey to Empowered Health

As you reach the final pages of your
Balance Life Pharmacist Medical Journal,
Take a moment to celebrate the progress you've made.
This journal was designed to help you:
Track your symptoms, medications, and treatments clearly
Prepare for doctor visits with confidence and clarity
Capture questions, labs, and insights that matter
Reflect on your goals, emotions, and well-being
Bridge traditional and natural healing approaches
Your voice matters. Your health is personal.
By using this journal, you've taken a powerful step toward
becoming your own best advocate.
Keep this journal close, bring it to appointments, and
continue writing your health story with
courage, grace, and intention.

Remember: wellness is not a destination—it's a daily practice.

With gratitude and strength,
Jill Johnson, RPh

Founder, Balance Life Pharmacist

www.balanceliferx.com | @BalanceLifePharmacist |
admin@balanceliferx.com
(248) 786-9422

ABOUT THE PUBLISHER

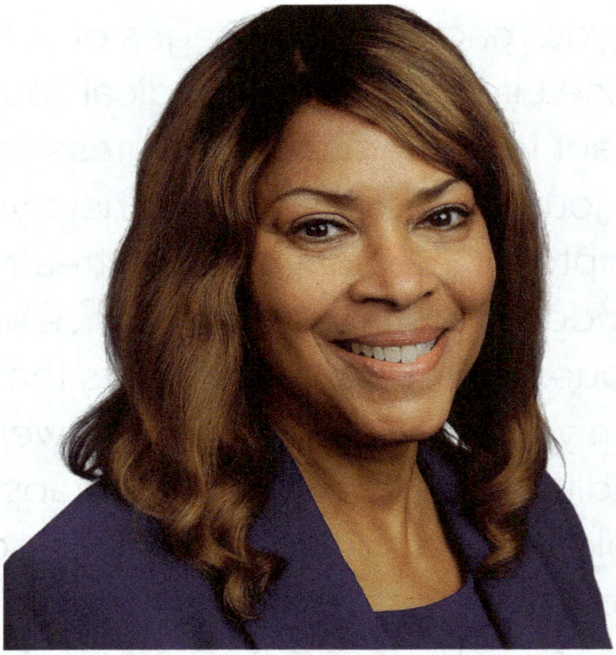

As a Pharmacist and a Social Entrepreneur, Jill Johnson has dedicated over 30+ years to the field of pharmacy, combining her extensive professional experience with a deep passion for holistic lifestyle and healing. As a long-time advocate for homeopathic medicine, she has made it her mission to empower others with natural, effective approaches to wellness. With a heart for healing and a commitment to lifelong learning, Jill brings both warmth and wisdom to her work. She is the mother of two adult children and enjoys traveling and developing affordable housing in her community.

www.ingramcontent.com/pod-product-compliance
Lightning Source LLC
LaVergne TN
LVHW060044210926
848481LV00013B/3952